From
MESS
to
MESSAGE

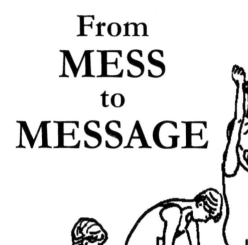

Understanding the hidden healing messages behind
pain and suffering

Cleo Darcia Graham

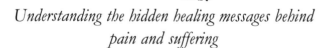

Published by
Thorton Publishing, Inc.
303-794-8888
www.ProfitablePublishing.net
17011 Lincoln Ave. #408
Parker, Colorado 80134

Edited by Essentials Educational Services and Products
P.O. Box 2464
Springfield, MA 01109-2464
http://www.eesplus.com

Cover Design Diane Bilal
Spirit of Words
New Haven, CT
dianebilal@aol.com

Cover Layout
EJ Thornton
Thornton Publishing, Inc.

ISBN: 1-932344-89-6
www.BooksToBelieveIn.com/Inspirational.php

Praise God,
from
Whom All Blessings Flow

Dedicated to

My parents
Mary and the late James Ingram
who taught me how to live
above my pain and suffering.

My husband, Melvin H. Graham
my love and my friend

Our sons,
Melvin R. and Justin H.
who remind me that "It's all good."

"He reveals deep and hidden things;
He knows what is in the darkness, and light dwells with Him."

Daniel 2:22

Contents

Acknowledgements
Introduction

Contents

Acknowledgements

All praises are due to God.

I would like to thank all of you for your prayers, love and support. If I have failed to acknowledge you by name, please know my heart sincerely appreciates your efforts on my behalf. Much thanks to you all:

Melvin H., my wonderful husband, and our sons, Melvin R. and Justin H., for their unconditional love, patience, and support throughout this journey.

Reena Duhamel for her kindness and for sharing with me, Mya, my precious granddaughter.

Mary and the late James Ingram, my parents, whose love has nurtured the depths of my soul.

Renay Ingram, teacher, and Diane Makini Bilal, artist, my sweet sisters, who believed in and encouraged me while sharing their talents in order to support my endeavor to complete this book.

James Ingram, my brother, who encourages me in his own special way, and my precious mother-in-law Cora Graham and sisters-in-law Gwendolyn Graham and Mary Anderson.

My aunt Mamie Saulsbury, Oni, Tamu, and Mansour, and all of my other relatives too numerous to mention.

Pauline Harvey Covington, my beloved friend and spiritual sister,
Lee Varella, my dear friend and "big sister,"
Dolores Norton Braica, my devoted friend, and my loyal friend, Christine Murphy.

Rev. Eleanor Naomi Craig, my spiritual mother, whose constant love and prayers have nourished me. Much love to Donna O'Connor and the NC100BW - RI "Queens".

Carolyn Addison and Ann McGloshen, my prayer partners, Dr. Dolores Seymour whose positive energy is truly contagious.

Much love to my "cheerleaders" Marjorie Petrucelli, Judy Smith DePerla, Sheila Brown, Cheryl Fitzgerald, Teruko Langwell, Penny Shar, Evelyn Cooley, Reina Avila, Alice Cashill, and all my Aqua Aerobic friends at the Sherwood Health Club.

Dr. Leah Adams, Dr. Vlad Zayas, Sue Rodrigues, Dr. Pradeep Chopra, Dr. Mindy Rosenbloom, Rebecca Gesson, and chiropractors Dr. Joyce Martin and Dr. Hogan-Casey, my great medical team.

Dr. Dawna Blake, Cindy Tibert, Richard Nerenberg and all my other co-workers who never forget about me.

Attorney Katherine Smith, you are an angel.

Pastor Theresa Smith of Bethel AME Church for her intercessory prayers.

To my dear church family, the Olney Street Baptist Church, Reverends Arnett Fugett, Dr. Perry Alexander, and Women's Ministry for keeping the 'light' in my heart burning.

Finally, Michael Poulin for his patience, and Dr. Mamie Oliver for leading me to EJ at Thornton Publishing. I am grateful for all that you have done to make this book possible.

A Note from a Dear Friend

Dear Cleo,

Thank you for the opportunity to preview this book and witness the evolution of your spiritual journey. You have demonstrated that to enjoy the sweet fragrance of roses you may have to endure the pain of the thorny stems.

Continue to trust God and to know that His Blessing is upon you.

Love,
Pauline Harvey Covington, RN, BSN
Research Nurse Supervisor / Coordinator

Introduction

What if your life was changed by a sudden injury or illness?
What if you asked God to heal you, to make you well, to help you get through the pain and suffering?
What if He answered, but not in the way that you expected?

This is my story; however, it could also be your story. If you or a loved one has experienced pain and suffering, we may share a common bond between us - especially if it was triggered by a sudden and unexpected event that was beyond your control.

I was at the crest of my nursing career and had a fine reputation as a Nurse Practitioner and as a person who enjoyed my work as well as new challenges. I successfully worked in medical clinics at a busy hospital where I always gave my best; at times I felt indispensable. Suddenly, my whole life changed dramatically when I injured my back while examining a patient in a clinic. The pain immediately ripped across my back and down my legs. The next day, the pain was so excruciating that I could barely walk. I was certain that it was more than a simple backache. I began treatment in a hospital emergency room and subsequently required continued medical care.

Although I was medicated and on bed rest, I was alert enough to pray and meditate as I had done for years. The difference was that I was held captive by my physical condition and it was during this time that my spiritual connection to God grew stronger. The Spirit of God spoke and I listened more intently than ever before. Suddenly, the messages began to come to me in a flurry and I became spiritually and mentally filled. I felt like I would burst open and could hardly contain the thoughts imprinted on my mind. Through this inspiration, I began to write, as I believed that the Spirit of the Lord spoke to me. There were days I had nothing to write about, but there was never a day that I did not feel God's presence. He sent angels to me in the form of my family, friends, coworkers and strangers, all for the Divine purpose of helping me to heal.

During those times when I was discouraged due to unrelenting and intense back pain, I was inspired by these biblical passages:

"The Lord is my light and my salvation; whom shall I fear? The Lord is the strength of my life; of whom shall I be afraid?"
Psalm 27:1

"Be still, and know that I am God: I will be exalted among the heathen, I will be exalted in the earth."
Psalm 46:10.

"Ye shall not need to fight in this battle: set yourselves, stand ye still and see the salvation of the Lord with you..."
2 Chronicles 20:17.

"He that dwelleth in the secret place of the most High shall abide under the shadow of the Almighty."
Psalm 91:1

"Surely goodness and mercy shall follow me all the days of my life: and I will dwell in the house of the Lord for ever."
Psalm 23:6

Comforted by these words, I began to slowly learn to live outside of the pain and suffering that had consumed my life. I wrote about issues, events, and people who were also coping with pain and suffering related to illnesses, disappointments, and losses. Poetically, I described some of the remedies such as water aerobics, bible study, rest, relaxation breathing, prayer, positive life skills, physical therapy, spine injection treatments, medication, nutrition, acupuncture, stretches, devices, Reiki, and writing that have been a part of my goal towards recovery. I asked God for answers and He responded-not always in the ways that I had expected.

Once, while I was a visitor at a church service, a very compassionate minister laid her hands on me during a healing prayer for those in attendance. I was convinced more than ever that I was on the path to healing. By midweek, during aqua pool therapy, I listened as a trauma survivor recounted her near-death experience after a car accident that resulted in multiple injuries. She stated that she clung to life holding the arm of a Medic Rescuer. She said that she felt as if her life was slipping away - so, she touched his arm in order that she could feel life. Now, her life has more meaning - she says that she has God to thank for sending her an angel at that critical time.

By Friday of that week, I had a Reiki treatment by Donna James, RN, who is a very warm-spirited person. She touched my heart and my soul. I felt the presence of God working through her during this treatment at her home. Although I was not pain free, I felt good when I left her. The following day, my husband, my fourteen-month old granddaughter, and I traveled to Boston, Massachusetts for my appointment with an Asian physician who is board certified in family medicine, acupuncture, and herbal medicine. That visit joined the Eastern and Western philosophies of healing together into one for me. I often struggled between both of these distinct worlds as far as integrating the respective medical therapies. Fortunately, this medical appointment in Boston happened at a time when I had very few options due to the side effects of my medications. I experienced short-term relief and optimism after that visit.

Over the next several months, I had various non-surgical treatments in an effort to heal my injured back and to restore my overall health.   Time, prayer, water exercises, committed medical providers, and love from my family and friends have helped me immensely during this time.

You might ask, as I have so many times, "Why should I bear so much pain and suffering?" There is a story to tell. Read and discover, as I have, these hidden healing messages from God. Let me share with you poetically what I have discovered through pain and suffering.

Chapter 1

Planting

"I   (Paul) planted, Apollos watered,
but God gave me the increase."

1 Corinthians 3:6

Pain

The pain won't let me go.
But I said, "Pain!
God is going to have His way
So you might as well sit down.
You know you're too weak to fight with God."

I'll just stand right behind Him
and faithfully watch what He does to you.

Watch out! I got my shoes on,
I'm heading out the door.

That back pain is not going
to hold me back anymore.

Listening to Me

I'm not sleepy, just tired
Eyes closed, deep breathing
Listening to the sounds of silence
Things…
I hear the floor creak
I hear the birds speak
I hear the cars drive by
I hear the trees shiver
The little baby cry
I hear the dog bark
I hear the mailman park

I'm not sleeping
Got my eyes closed, tired
Body still, mind at peace
Listening to silence
Listening to me.

Attitude

Your attitude
is what frames everything you do.
Imagine having a beautiful
picture in an old rugged frame-
A frame which is broken, cracked, dusty,
and filled with grime and mildew.

Much like our attitude,
we can allow a build up of hurt.
Disappointments and fear to settle in
and build up layers of debris.
This will eventually affect our approach,
not only to our everyday life events,
but cloud our approach to new
and positive opportunities.

Therefore, we need to periodically
dust off, clean and polish our frames anew.
So we may view the beauty of
our picture, framed, in a clear bright
and positively inviting attitude.

Our Hands

Our hands can touch, rub, hold and scold
Our hands can heal, peel, manipulate and steal
Our hands can pray, say I love you in more than one way
Our hands can clap and rock a baby on our lap
Our hands can do almost anything
Depending on our thoughts and functioning.

Our hands can be God's hands wrapped up in love
Responding only to directions from above
Our hands can warm a cold and broken heart
Hold a tearful face whose life has fallen apart.

Our hands can speak the truth about our roots
Show compassion for us, too long overdue
Our hands can come together and shake for peace
Or stand alone, one gun, one hand, on a trigger to release.

Our hands can pass on a virulent disease
Or hold it in tissue when we cough or sneeze
Our hands can build monuments mountains high
Our hands can rise up, fly airplanes in the sky.

Our hands can speak for peace louder than we sing
Our hands can give God thanks for everything.

Live and Learn

The longer I live
the more I learn...
That sweetness and kindness
are not imaginary things
That music and birds
are not only what we hear and sing
That you can have love
without knowing where it begins
That you can feel comfort,
warmth and relief within.

The longer I live,
the more broader my steps
Have memory of places
not traveled to yet
I have friends in high places
Loved ones of all kinds
Have grace, joy and mercy
The best friends you can find.

War

Are we at war with ourselves or them?
Our egos, indecision, points, counter points, no end
They get larger
Farther and further
Peace can't win
It's destroyed in our minds
Before the war begins
Tell me who are we fighting?
It's the battle within
Our borders, ourselves
To feel free again
If I kick a can
Does it mean I won't feel pain,
Does it mean that the can won't roll back again
To hit me in my foot, trip me, cause a sprain?
Surprise attack all over again
Can peace have the final say?
Who are we at war with
Ourselves or them today?

How Much Pain Is Fear?

My fear is that fear
will come in like a thief in the night
and steal our joy, replace it with fright

By morning we will awaken
in a deep dark haze,
We won't know what we've lost
or what can be saved
We will be startled by every sound feeling
like danger is all around

Every man is suspect
Paranoia abound
We will be tied up like ships,
too afraid to sail free
We'll forget God is the vine
and we are branches of His tree
If we would just hold on
Hang in there you'll see
The fear will be lifted if we only believe.

How's the Weather Outside?

(In memory of my grandmother, Momma)

I wonder if my 100-year-old grandmother
asked that question each time to find out what
we visitors went through to get to her:

"How's the weather outside?"

"Oh, Momma!
The weather is cold,
its windy but the snow is melting"

"Oh, Momma!
It's hot outside
The sweat is pouring off of our faces"

"Oh, Momma!
It's raining so hard it looks
Like everyone is crying
Tears of joy and tears of sorrow."

You've gone on to heaven
To be with your Lord,
"Oh, Momma!
"How's the weather outside there?"

"Chile' the sun is shining."
There's flowers everywhere
The weather's nice here"
"Oh yeah? Hush your mouth."

Don't Blame Me

Don't be so eager to blame
For all your trials
Your shame
You clearly knew the game
But continued to do the same
Not caring about the family name
You did it over and over again
Now you're left with years of pain
What did you really gain?
More money, prestige you claim?
And now you're alone
No one came
To bail you out - it's insane
The price you paid for fame
Because living life your way was in vain
Don't blame me for your pain.

Me, Myself, and I
(Is Three Really Company?)

Picture yourself looking in the mirror.
There's a little girl who is hungry
and asking to be picked up, hugged and loved.
Take her home with you.
Give her a warm bath.
Smooth warm oil on her face, hands, back and feet
paying attention to every detail of her fingers and toes.
Now cover her in soft cotton pajamas
and fluffy slippers.
Sit across from her at the table and serve her
warm soup and nicely warmed bread and butter.
Observe her smile as she enjoys the attention
she is receiving from you.
Acknowledge her thanks to you and her thanks to God
for you finding her at home with herself.
You are feeling at home with you.
YOU ARE SHE.
You tuck yourself in for a peaceful sleep
looking forward to another day
and another look in the mirror
A CLEARER VIEW OF YOU!

Baby Shoes

Baby shoes
Can I tip toe around the room?
Stretch my hands out
Touch yours, too?

Baby shoes
Teach me how to run and fly
May I walk alone?
At least try?

Baby shoes
Makes me want to dance real hard
Shake my hips
and move my thighs

Baby shoes
Soft and white as snow

Baby shoes
Never will get old

I'll wear my baby shoes
my whole life through

My sweet soft baby shoes
I'll never let go of you.

From Mess to Message

I was the youngest girl of four
In a bottom double bunk
One room
Four kids
Who snored and feet stunk
Lesson: I learned to live with people in small funky places
We used the same cloth to wash our faces
I was the third one in line
I was left with smears and messes

I was three
by the time I climbed a tree
Running from a squirrel
I scraped my knee
Lesson: I learned don't waste time running from something that's
not chasing you

I was five
when I learned how to dive
Except we had no pool
My forehead split open wide
Lesson: I learned to look and think before jumping in

I was seven
when I learned about heaven
I prayed to go there
when in trouble, lonely or in fear
Lesson: Be careful what you pray for - you might just get it

I was eleven
when I got my first job
I scrubbed floors with a bucket

and rags bent down on all fours
Lesson: Come prepared and use your own equipment

I was sixteen
when I sold shoes
Handling so many feet, smelling
I refused to wear the very shoes
I was selling
Lesson: Do what you believe to be right for you

I was seventeen
when I worked as an aid in a nursing home
I thought I caught every disease known
Lesson: Never work in a job that makes you feel sicker than
those you're caring for

I was eighteen
when I went to college
and had a job shelving books
That's when I met my husband
falling off the chair when we looked
Lesson: Looks can be deadly, just a quick glimpse first

I was twenty-two
and a nurse when I murmured "I do"
I was sure it was like our dating,
besides, what else was left to do
Lesson: Know, plan, commit, love and have fun

I was twenty-four
when my first one was born
I held him so much from morning to dawn
He soon had the feeling he was part of my arm
Lesson: Don't hold too much, too tight, don't overdo

I was twenty-five
when we bought our first house
We had no money left to even buy a couch
Lesson: If you bite off more than you can chew, your faith in
God will see you through

I was twenty-eight
when my period was late
I knew I was pregnant and had a November due date
He delivered a week early all to my surprise
I didn't even have time to finish cooking my French fries
Lesson: Never start anything you can't finish

Now I am forty-eight
A grandma of a great big girl named Mya Justina
She's sweet and neat
At ten months she hugs, kisses and hollers
She likes us to tickle her feet
and giggles just like her father
She loves to hold hands walking
from room to room
When she is at my house, that's a workout
that's not over soon
Lesson: This is time well spent - enjoy

Approaching fifty
in a few months
I've been forced to slow down, rest, recuperate and chill
I'm finding more pennies on the ground
Lesson: Be alert to the changing seasons all
around and within you.
LOOK FOR THE PENNIES FROM HEAVEN
REMINDING US that IN GOD WE TRUST..

God, I Thank You

Lord,
I stand here on my own two feet
My hands are open
For you I greet
My head bowed down
My mind is free
'Cause I'm so glad
For another day to see
Your marvelous works
Your grace and mercies
I raise my hands above the earth
To spread Your word like seeds in dirt
The power of Your word
Gives me light
As I pray to you
Morning noon and night
I pray You'll keep me in Your sight
Protect me and guide me
With You everything's alright.

Must I Die Before I Live?

I mustn't die before I live
or I will miss my chance to give
a part of me I held onto so long

Waiting for my name to be called

I'm waiting!
Think they'll call me next?
But what if my name is not on the list

I wanted to hear my name
called out loud
so that when I performed
my friends would be proud

It's getting late
and seems it doesn't matter
I'll call my own name,
give my part and leave right after

It's no big deal
whether they scream, shout or holler
I did my part and I don't even want a dollar
Now I can live my life
because I gave before I die
I'm applauding myself so hard I could cry.

Who Turned Off the Light?

Who turned off the light?
I know that it's daytime but it looks like it's night
The shadows have fallen on faces so grim
I wonder if we will ever see sunshine again

Who turned off the light?
My spirit is grieving, my body's uptight
I suddenly forgot which switch is the light
One flick and I got it, but that's not all true
The power is missing - the connection is too

Who turned off the lights ?
What am I to do in the dark
The answer I'm told
is in the books of Matthew and Mark
I must love the Lord with all my mind, soul, strength and heart
Prayer and true faith will turn darkness into light

Who turned the light off?
My connection to Thee
was suddenly broken because
I ignored God's teachings.

Rivers of Thoughts

These thoughts are like rivers
flowing through my mind
How can I explain it
when I don't have the time
My mind keeps on racing
My pen runs out of ink
I'm so filled with spirit
I can't even think
The messages are clearly imprinted
before my eyes
If my hands would write faster
than the words I see pass by
In my mind there's an urgency
that time's running out
I mustn't stop here
There's still more to talk about
The feelings seem useless
but then these are thoughts
I don't have control of, it must be the Lord
Is trying to tell me slow down, listen carefully
I've been trying to tell you how to be free
From worry and pain, disappointment, and shame
This is not some kind of psychic or a silly game
The message is simple
It's fully guaranteed
You must pray, give, love, have faith, believe
and follow Me.

Whose Shoulder Shall I Cry On?

Whose shoulder shall I cry on?
When I'm on bended knees
Praying
"Oh Lord have mercy on me"

My mother is sickly, my father passed on
My sisters are busy, my brother's mind half gone

Whose shoulder shall I cry on?
When I'm on bended knees
Praying
"Oh Lord have mercy on me"

My husband's at home but, he's so hard to see
My sons are invisible or they pretend to be
My friends often call, send cards, flowers, candy
My Pastor and Deacons gave communion and prayed for me

Whose shoulder shall I cry on?
When I'm on bended knees
To God be the glory
Cry on HIS shoulder indeed.

Putting Up with Putting Out

Everyone wants you when you're putting out fires in their life
Working hard, making money, making peace, settling strife
When you're broken and broke hungry as you could be
No one knocks on your door to give you any relief
But my souls at peace and my spirit is free
God has shined His Light on me
Shown favor, gives me victory
My patience is never thin
I believe in Him
If I put up

or put out

doesn't

matter

He's

my

friend

until

the

end.

Gone but Not Forgotten

By the time I blinked
you were gone
By the time I breathed
you were not here
I can hardly think how life would be without you now
The flame that took you out burns in my soul
You were just here
So very dear to our hearts
Now we're apart
Doesn't matter whose fault
You're not here
for me to say I love you in so many ways
But I'm here to show the world
you are still loved today
I know you see the love and feel our pain
But one day we'll meet again
Sorry I wasn't there to shelter you from the storm
Wasn't there to keep you from all harm
I'm writing this song to let you know
I loved you then
I love you now
I'll love you always.

In His Care

Need to get a lot of loving care
Need to be around people who share
the love and compassion you once gave
Now that you're gone I'm all alone
there's nothing to say
But I loved you more than life oh yeah
Many dreams came true when I was with you
Now you're gone and I'm all alone
But you said we'd never part,
We'll always be together in our hearts
You said right from the start to pray
Said God will always help you find the way
To heal a broken heart, when things fall apart
Remember when we stopped, parked
Closed our eyes took deep breaths in the dark
Remember Light came in and you said
it was the Spirit of God our friend
We mustn't fear just let Him in
And we did that night
Now I'm trying with all my might
Because you're not here tonight
But I hear the Spirit telling me everything is all right
I feel the same peace I felt that night in the park
Remembering when Light came in
You said it was the spirit of God, our friend
We mustn't fear just let Him in
And we did that night
Although you're gone away
I can feel His presence and yours every day
I really miss holding you but, I feel your spirit

Because it warms my heart even though we're apart
Everything's going to be all right
I let the Light shine in
Now my joy and strength
comes from within
I'll always miss you
You showed me that God is my friend
and with us until the end.

We Are Just Seeds

Aren't we all like little seeds
Born to help someone in need
Knowing that some day we will be planted in the ground
But before that time we will travel around
At times we will be carried by an insect
or moved by a forceful breeze
No matter how we get there you see
Our purpose is to spread joy, peace and harmony
As a seed we can be that hope
For those who are struggling and can't cope
The seeds of love, kindness, compassion
Unfortunately not all seeds travel the same road
Not all seeds do good deeds
At the end of life, the seed is planted in the ground
Waiting to bloom
Only you decide what flower will burst through
It may be a weed or a beautiful rose
Only you can decide how your seed grows.

Mother Wit
(My mother's advice about terrorism)

I will not buy bottled water, duct tape or a roll of plastic
Says mother wit
Ignorance has nothing to do with it

I will not fear, run away, and think about what if
It has nothing to do with what I have or get
Says mother wit

Apathy has not stolen my appetite for worry
I'm just not going to prematurely feel sorry
Says mother wit

If it's my time to go and God knows I've done my best
Then it must be my time to take a long soft rest
Says mother wit

"The Bible says: if God is for you who can be against you,"
Now that's a fact
Bottled water, duct tape and plastic won't stand up to that
Says mother wit

I'm going to keep on living, praying 'till its time to quit
My faith and trust in God will protect me
I'm not worried the least bit.

Shall I Complain or Withstand the Pain?

I'm not one to complain
But I'm really in pain
Yet, I look for many thanks
It helps my mind not go blank
Slows the pain down
Takes away my frown
I'm thankful for this time
To write a song or rhyme
'Cause without this time you see
I'd never know my capabilities
Lying flat, lying still
Wanting to help you instead of me
Not feeling comfortable resting peacefully
Knowing, rest and patience are my friends
Certainly not my enemy
I must learn to slow down
I must let go of people who put me down
I must not let their selfish words get me down
There's much more pain when you fall down
However, for my own healing
I must lie down
Keep my prayers up
Wait and watch for blessings to come down.

Who Is Your Boss?

What if God is your boss?
You could not deny the cross
That Jesus
Suffered
Died
Rose
To save our weary souls

If God is your boss
Why do you roam around so lost?
Worried
Troubled
Buying
Psychic solutions at a high cost

If God is your boss
Then you should work for Him
Doing all things for His glory
Our Savior
Our Lord
Our Friend.

Pain,
Why Must You Come Back Again?

Pain,
Why must you come back again?
I thought that Comfort was your friend
You were not with me through the night
But early this morning you returned to fight
A battle to keep me filled with tears, uptight

Pain,
You cannot control my mind or my body
I'll say a prayer, take these pills, you'll be sorry
'Cause I'm not giving in
or giving up, you can't stop me
I have much to do

Pain,
You're not my destiny
Oh Comfort and Peace are here
and they brought Joy with them too
So, get out of town

Pain,
There's no room for you.

Assignment Confinement

My assignment is a forced confinement
to slow down, heal, reflect
Get a lifestyle alignment
Think about why I do what I do
and who is it serving
God or you

My mind wonders about the end result
Will it matter if I do it or don't
All the fuss and movement with no rest in between
Makes me feel like I'm losing a battle with me
because my mind is racing
with my body and spirit wants to be free

My soul doesn't want any of this anxiety
As I lay here in confinement
Pain and weakness hold me down
I am now captive and attentive
to what changes I must make now
Free my spirit
Let my soul be strengthen
My body and my mind, all for God's glory.

Home Sweet Home

When you're at home for a long rest
Instead of seeing one ant you see many piled up in a mess
You now see lots of dust in your house
It didn't matter when you were moving about
But now it looks like you're about to move out

Dishes piled high, dirty clothes, and wet ones, no room to dry
Pillows flat, from lying so long on my back
Pain is creeping down my leg
I'm hungry - sure wish I had a scrambled egg

Whoever is home is still asleep
I don't see any movement or hear a peep
My sisters say I must concentrate on getting well
I must not let troubles or worries interfere with my health

Physically, mentally, spiritually
I must heal and renew my energy
As things pile up and bills are paid late
I can't let that interfere with healing
It can all wait

But I can't wait to pray each and every day
God gives me strength and peace
Blesses me with these words and has mercy on me
As I crawl out of bed stretch my spine
Relax my mind…A new day has begun
Surprise to find all chores have been done

The coffee is perking; the eggs and toast are still warm
The house smells so clean, my worries are none
Who did all this and when?
What happened? Why? It doesn't matter
Just know that God's angels have moved in.

Chapter 2

Watering

"So then neither he who planteth is any
thing, neither he that watereth,
but God that giveth the increase."

1 Corinthians 3:7

Fighting Back With Water

When I first met instructor Pam
It was in a pool of warm water
All I knew how to do was smile
But my back ached so much that smiling didn't matter
As I paddled my way
Arms stretched reaching for the sky
What was I doing in this sea of strange smiling faces and why

"Smile," Pam said. "Do it mindfully
Pull your belly in
Flatten your back
Raise your arms
Do your jumping jacks
Bend your knees
Don't forget to deep breathe
Go with the flow
Turn around against it
Keep on moving
Don't quit
Elongate your neck
Parallel your chin…"

Thank God for healing
So feel good deep within.

Don't Ask What?

Don't ask to be lied to
Just don't ask
Then, you'll never know what's true
If you ask then
Be prepared
To get a lie or maybe the truth
You won't have to worry
You won't feel the pain
If you just don't ask
the questions again.

Get Out of God's Way

Get out of God's way
So He can work on you today

Stop, sit, and breathe quietly
Focus your mind
Relax your body

Surrender all thoughts
Do not speak
Get out of God's way
Make the road easy

For Him to get to you
Through you
Abide in you
Therefore, you can feel his presence
You can hear His truths.

On the Eve of War

First, I heard the dog howl
Then I heard the fly buzz
and I heard the bird knock on my window
Heard you whisper in my ear
What are you all telling me?
Is it something I long to hear?

I can hear footsteps rushing by
I can hear the sound of planes in the sky
Telephones ringing, I hear kisses and long goodbyes
What are they all trying to tell me and why?

I can hear the sound of rain
I hear laughter and cries of pain
I hear the prayers of a young child
Bring my daddy home again
I can hear cheers of joy
I hear the sound of a broken toy

Then I can hear a heart beat fade
I can hear people praying and songs of praise
I can hear you say it's alright
I can hear messages as clear as candlelight
I can hear your breathing so calm serene
I can hear your hands gently stroking me

I can hear the sounds of distress, pain, love and harmony
I can hear the messages of peace,
I hear the ticking of the clock
I can hear whispers and war talk
I can hear these sounds on the eve of war
What are they telling me and why?

Healing Thoughts

My mind says I am healed
My body just does not know it
My faith says be healed
My prayers say believe it
My soul says healing starts within
My peace says to begin
My spirit says don't give up or give in
God says be patient
I'm here to help you again and again.

Climb Back Inside Your Body

Climb back inside your body
What is it that you see?
A tug of war between two people
Struggling to be free
Look closely
What do you find in your mind?
Is it cluttered?
Is it closed?
Is it open?
Do you know?
Take a look at your eyes
Do you see love and truth?
Are your eyes open?
Closed?
Do you have faith without proof?
Are your eyes warm?
Are they kind?
Reflection of your mind?
Pay attention to your mouth
and the words you speak so clear
Sending spirit filled messages
or just words polluting the air?
Touch your heart and feel each beat
Feel blood flowing through and through
Nourishing, renewing, sustaining the life in you
Is what you see within you the same as what they see?
An open mind?
A clean heart?
Clear eyes
A mouth pure?
A spirit of love?
A peaceful soul?
A blessed life for sure.

Look at Yourself

Look at yourself against the backdrop of the sun
What a beautiful flower you have become
Arms stretched so wide like gorgeous flower petals
Colors make me feel good, even makes me smile a little
Your fragrance so sweet
Like ripe mangos from a tree
So soft, so smooth
I feel like hugging me
Because you held on through the storm
Stood upright in the rain
You kept growing and growing
Despite the pain
When people trampled on you
Tore your leaf, crushed your stem
You kept your roots deeply planted
Intact within
You looked up to the sky
The sun shined down on your face
Thanking God for placing you
at this time in this place
New leaf and new stem,
New arms and strong spine
Yet, what matters most is what's on your mind
Not what's clinging to you
like insects or dew on a vine
Either way it's fine it's time
For you to blossom and renew
Spring forth
Bend forward
Palms up toward the sun,
Inhale spirit
A new day has begun.

All for Peace

Let peace pour down
like a gentle summer rain
Let peace flow like rivers of blood
flowing through our veins
Let peace shine on us
like the rays of the sun
Let peace come to us to each and everyone
Let peace move in us
in our thoughts and every mindful deed
Let peace rule in us for this is truly what we need
Let peace stand before us

with an open hand and heart
Let peace be with us
let it be here from the start.

What's the Worst That Could Happen?

What's the worst that could happen
if we stand, cup our hands and pray
or fold our hands, get on our knees and say
Father we need your help today?

What's the worst that could happen
if we faced east or west
bowed our heads, covered or undressed,
looked down or up instead
prayed our best and let God do the rest?

What's the worst that could happen
if our hands touched and our words spoke of unity
if our lives bind together like a fine silky thread
not torn, connected instead?

What's the worst that could happen
if we stopped pretending we don't need each other
stopped killing our spirits, murdering our souls,
start loving one another?

What's the worst that could happen
if we said a little prayer,
a gentle breath, a silent moment,
allowing spirit in?

What's the worst that could happen
if we prayed together, no matter how far or near?

What's the worst that could happen
if we showed each other we care.

Today I Heard You Say

Today I heard You say
you must have faith and be obedient
Humble yourself,
Always pray and
Be willing to wash feet
I heard You say,
that I'm the salt of the earth,
You anointed my head with oil.

I heard You say,
to purify myself in the coolness of water
You told me angels will be sent my way
Just trust and believe, never cease to pray.

Today, I listened.
Today, I walked the swimming pool
A friendly stranger named Dolores walked with me too
She took me to the steam room
which was filled with a sweet fragrance
and warm stones caressing the water
that bounced against it like a dance.

She rubbed a poultice of coarse salt
and oil into my feet
I felt Your Calming Spirit move from her to me
I felt Your healing power.

I heard You clearly speak
through another lady who said to me,
"You're walking better, more upright
You're going to be alright."

I heard You speak these words of comfort
I never asked to see Your face
Today I heard You say
you must be obedient,
humble enough to wash feet,
have faith, pray and seek You every day.

Pray for All

As we bow our heads and pray for you
we pray for our enemies too
That we might all ask for peace, equality
that justice, kindness, sincere desire to be free
of greed, hatred, strife and misery.

So when you pray, pray for all of us
All who are fighting
All who are defending,
All who are wounded, captive, missing,
dead or alive

Pray for all mankind
God wants all of us.
Each and everyone,
To extend our prayers
Spread our hands
Reaching each soul one by one
To pray, pray, pray until peace is won
Pray for one and pray for all
This is truly God's call.

Slippery Slope

Today I feel like I'm on a slippery slope
At times being propelled forward, full of hope
At times sliding downward, can hardly cope
with the physical pain yet not as intense
As the mental anguish of so much dependence
on others good will, kindness, as well as my own common sense
Which at times is fading when I pretend to be
full of strength and energy

Then my movements jolt my memory,
Reminding me of my pain reminding me of my disability
A temporary challenge, not an impossibility
forces me to change my life but keep intact
my feelings and spirituality

I must reach for you in a different way
You mustn't hold me so tight around my waist
I must stand tall
Don't let my chin fall to my chest
Tighten my abdomen, relax all the rest
Move with me, let's dance
Give me a second chance
to feel the rhythm in my body
passing through the pain
Making me feel alive again
Although I must take steady and deliberate steps
I can keep up the pace, now is no time to rest
'cause I can still whisper in your ear, kiss your lips,
touch you and know that I am blessed.

Can You Make Peace Without Causing Pain?

War
Is it one big whiteout or an eraser smear?
Wiping out what was once there
Shoving our way of peace down their throats
Making who ever remain speechless
and without much hope
for their own sanity,
their own way to live free
Thinking for them
Making decisions
Planning strategies
all in the name of peaceful harmony.

A Not So Imaginary Friend

A
Not so imaginary friend
That's what God is to me
He is with me from the beginning to the end
With me when I fall
With me whenever I call
A
Not so imaginary friend
Loves me unconditionally
Sees my faults
Sees my weaknesses
But doesn't desert me
My
Not so imaginary friend
so gentle, loving and kind
My
Not so imaginary Friend
Sends angels to me every time
When I have a need or have troubles on my mind
I thank
My
Not so imaginary Friend
Thank you God for the hope and help you send.

My First Love
(Inspired after reading Psalm 63:1-8)

My First Love is for God
Everything and everyone will one day disappear
But God's love will always be near
Here with me
Present
Always touching my life
Anointing my head
Coming to me in the form of a cool breeze
Or a soft flickering light like a candlewick at night
His daily presence is shown
Through so many people unknown
Angels with invisible halos and wings
Letting me know they're here
Because when my ears ring
They surround me but do not smother me
Pave the way
Clear my path
Whisper to me, "it's okay"
Because God my first love is here everyday
No need to worry
Come what may
I hear your voice in the depths of a crowd
I see you in many places and on many faces
I can feel your touch holding me rocking me
Supplying my every need
Thank you God
You are my first love
You are my King.

What Should I Say
and How Shall I Think?

Say nothing
Just think good thoughts
Conversations within
Between you and me
Silent gestures
Face to face our eyes meet
Yet, we look but do not speak
My mind continues the conversation within
A strong dialogue searching for answers
Finding comfort just being
Always in God's presence
So joyfully I sing
Praise and thanksgiving
For the risen King.

Can I Tell You About This Pain?

Can I tell you about this pain that crawls across my left spine
to my behind
Pours down my left leg
Give me a break I beg
As it travels to my knee
Down to my heel
Please let me be
I was so quiet in a restful sleep
Then the burning pain came and rescued me
From a period of tranquility
To a state of alert, wide awake
What is it I'm missing?
Why must I lay here and wait?
It must be time to medicate and meditate
Smooth cool thoughts running through my mind
Put out the fire down my spine
Find the path, I begin to feel relaxed
It's a wonderful feeling when the pain goes
So sweet so serene I can wiggle my toes
Focus my attention outside of myself
Look around, there's no one else
Here in the dark, late night hour
to celebrate my victory over pain's power.
As I fall off to a deep sound sleep
Thank you God
I am grateful indeed.

It Takes Two to Fly a Kite

It takes two to fly a kite
That is if your direction is right
Don't hold the string too tight
Let the wind push it beyond your height
Doesn't matter your strength or her might
If you do it right
You can fly a kite out of sight
But, it takes two to fly a kite
Lots of laughter keeps the spirit light
and easy
Now can't you see?
Flying a kite is a breeze.

God, Can I Move in with You?

For twelve weeks I was displaced
From the rush and rat race
Placed flat on my back, upright
Only to look side to side or up
To gaze upon Your face
was such a comforting sight

In times on my afflicted bed alone
I wait and wait
For Your marvelous healing
to deliver me from this state
Soon I realized not only must I wait,
I must move in with God
Let go, pack up, move forward, toward
A Higher place not in a physical sense
More of a spiritual reference

Urging me to place my trust in God above
Move on, move up and climb if you must
Slide back down, fall, but hold on and wait
Pray through it all
Know there's no problem too big or small
When you live with the Comforter,
you reside with a Holy Spirit
filled with peace, love and the Power to heal
So be encouraged, wait and pray
It's never more than you can bear
Stand still and wait
For the salvation of God is near.

Clipped Wings Will Fly Again

Clipped wings will fly again
Once more you are told to be still
Wait
Stand
Do nothing
It's not your battle
Win or lose you still must choose
To rest in faith
Pray
Trust the God who never looses
Must your wings be clipped to keep you here
Dwelling in His presence
Come close
Go near
But I can't do it you say
My wings are clipped, broken, I fear
I may never fly again that way
Clipped wings can fly again
Different stroke
Gliding high above the clouds
Resting on God's mercy
Bound to win
No doubt.

Quiet Suffering and Quiet Pain

Quiet Suffering
Quiet Pain
I can no longer think of myself
My miseries the same
When I think of how He suffered on the cross for us
It brings tears to my eyes
Yet a joy deep within
Quiet Suffering
Quiet Pain
I'm faced with my own cross to bear again.

Living on Pins and Needles

First there were pins
lots of them placed up and down my spine
acupuncture followed by deep penetrating massage
My back pain had control of my life
It dictated my every move and mood
like I was living in someone else's body
that was broken
so many thoughts and words unspoken
living on pins and needles
the medicine helped somewhat relieved
the pins and needle feeling down my leg
God comforted me when my mind
and heart felt pierced with pins and needles
Physical therapy,
water exercise,
whirlpool
epidural
injections too
prayers and chants,
family and friends
encouraging words
that it's okay
needless to say
it was all worth the joy I feel today.

Healing Heart, Thank You

Your sincere heart

helped to mend this broken body part

soothed this life that had fallen apart

fed a hungry soul starved
for love, peace and comfort

your heart so kind so sweet so loving so warm
your heart warmed my heart and made me feel calm

I thank you, thank God for you
from the depth of my heart to you

thank you for giving me a part of you

your heart so pure sincere and true
like an invisible healing balm felt in me through and through.

Attention!

Sit up and take notice
Pay attention
Concentrate
Focus
Look straight ahead
never mind what's behind
Press forward instead
Position your body
Align your head
Tune in
Inhale deep within
Now open wide
Allow spirit in
Feel the presence of Divine
Make up your mind
To take time
Slow down
Take a break
Don't wait until it's too late
Stop
Listen
Don't hesitate
Breathe deep
Feel the relief
Pay attention to peace.

Apart from You I Can Do Nothing

Apart From You I can do nothing
No matter how great or small
To You I owe it all
I take no credit
I accept all blame
Thank You for Your goodness
For forgiving all my shame
Can my eyes see without vision?
My mouth speaks without tongue or voice?
My ears hear without listening?
My hands touch without fingers to feel?
My feet carry me to and fro?
Apart from You I wouldn't know where to go.

Am I Productive?

I want to do something productive
Rest is productive
I want to be productive
Being faithful is productive
I want to accomplish so I can feel productive
Allowing healing is productive
I want to know that I am productive
Learning to rest and being still is productive
I want you to say that I'm productive
Not talking
Silent
Listening is productive
You are now more productive than you have ever been
You are just too busy worrying about it to notice.

On Her Way
(Dedicated to RI Superior Court Judge Rogeriee Thompson)

She's up north
She's a descendant of a slave
She's educated, polished, seasoned and brave
She's uniquely fashioned, home grown and God made
She's been in trouble, through trouble and fixed troubled souls
She's seen and heard more than you'd ever know
She's someone's wife, mother, sister, aunt and friend
She is a blessed woman
She's at times speechless
Yet her eyes speak loud and clear

She emanates simplicity, strength, beauty - far and near
She's patient, kind, she knows the path is not always bright
She's a judge - appointed not by civil right
but by her own might
She's not one to complain
Because their loss is her gain

She's gracefully disappointed and yet without shame
She's up north
Above it, physically, mentally, spiritually
She's on eagle's wings, rising
Flying above all their judgments
She's preoccupied with what God wants her to be.

Feed Me

Three little blackbirds hanging on a tree
One says, I see bread, will that lady feed me
Of course not, said one of the bird's buddy
Human beings must be told to give comfort, to share, to let go
That is why they can't fly, touch the sky, hold they're head high
Yes, they think they are the best,
think they're better than you and I
But, why are they lonely when there's so many of them
Because they really don't know how to be a true friend
You see, when we birds see bread or one small speck of food
We whistle to everyone out loud a sharp harmonious tune
We believe that there's always enough to go around
We don't worry about our next meal
or let problems get us down
Our faith foot steps forward,
keeps us balanced on God's ground.

Be Still While We Pray

Be still while we pray
Breathe in and out as you may
But be still as we pray
Cease conversing as there's nothing to say
When we turn ourselves to the Master to pray
Stand still
Stay, pray
Wait, watch,
We'll show you the way
Just stand
Sit and kneel
Cup hands,
Bowed heads
It's all okay
Just be still while we pray.

Thank You

Thank you
For each breath
Of air flowing in and out my nose

Thank you
For each heart beat
Blood of life from my head to toes

Thank you
For my hands
They move so efficient through each command

Thank you
For my feet
They allow me to stand

Thank you
For my eyes
They see Your wondrous works each day

Thank you
For my ears
They hear songs of praise and a quiet prayer

Thank you
For my mind
My soul, my life, and my spirit free
Thank you Lord - You have been so good to me.

Father's Day
(Dedicated to my late father James Ingram)

When you see a bird fly by
Hovering close over your head
When that bee buzzes at your window screen
Don't scream, let him in instead

When the light flickers
Or a deep soft whisper
makes you shiver
Close your eyes, smile, I'm here

When you have your doubts and worries
Confidence has run out
Remember what I taught you
What life is all about

You will succeed
if that's what you need
You will get through
When it's your time to

When you smell my after shave
and see the stuff that makes my hair behave
When you find my razor hairs in the sink
Just know that I am closer to you than you think

Close your eyes and dream of me
as often as you wish
Laugh and cry
as often as you reminisce

Although you buried me many days ago
There's a part of me that will never let go
Of the love I have for you my dear
Father's day is everyday and my love is sincere.

85

Crying in My Soup

Crying in my soup
Soaking my bread
Soggy fried fish won't do
Questions I don't have the answers to
How long?
Who knows the time frame?
Who knows when I'll have no pain?
Who knows when I can
Resume
Get on
Move on
Change
or return again

Crying in my soup
Wet napkins
Stained eyeglasses
the touch of a wet cheek
Dripping on my bread
Soggy fried fish
Oh how I wish

All this pain and worry were joy instead
It's enough to make you sad
It's plenty to make you weak
But not cause you to break
So let the tears fall
Until you get the call,
Maybe I'm too weak
Too tired to hold back
Just let go, relief, I'm not a perfect person

Crying in my soup
Soaking my bread
Soggy fried fish won't do
Questions I don't have the answers to ... how long?
Who knows the time frame?
Who knows when I'll have no pain?
Who knows when I can
Resume
Get on
Move on
Change
or return again.

Praying My Best Prayer

When I'm in pain
I pray my best prayer

"Lord have mercy
Shine your light
Relief is in sight"

When I'm in pain
I pray my best prayer

"Cool the burning
Smooth the aches,
So I no longer complain"

When I'm in pain
I pray my best prayer

"Come close
Come near
Your Hand on my hair
Let me touch You
or touch Your robe
You can heal me this I know"

When I'm in pain
I pray my best prayer

I find comfort
Love
Warmth
Relief
and answers
I find you near.

Thank You for the Hands

I thank you for the hands
that have touched me

I thank you for the hands
which have prayed for me

I thank you for the hands
which have massaged me

Manipulated me,
Pointed out to me
Directed me
Rested on me
Caressed me
Consoled me
Held me
Loved me
Hands
Which shake my hands
and my world.

What If Roses Could Talk?

This morning I cut off the neck of a rose.
Then I stuck it in a vase of bamboo shoots.
It happened when I rushed to close the door.
I didn't know, the rose, was peeking around the corner trying to
get a glimpse of my nose or maybe my toes.
I guess it was wondering
where was I rushing to on such a calm sunny day.
I was just barely out of bed. I washed up, dressed and prayed.
I never stopped to look and say,
"Oh, good morning rose. You smell so sweet today."
Your petals were open like they're ready to hug me.
But, I was too busy to hug you.
You see, I'm much too busy.
Then, the door slammed.
Looking back, I saw the rose's neck
crammed in between, inside and out.
as If it could shout, it would scream, "let me out."
In my haste, I ran back, no time to waste.
I kicked open the door.
The poor broken rose fell on the floor.
I picked it up.
I stuck it in a vase filled with water, rocks and a bamboo shoot.
Hoping it would grow new roots.
This morning in my haste, I cut off the neck of a rose.
This morning, I learned I must stop,
smell the roses, imagine the taste,
of a slower pace, perhaps a sweet embrace,
with roses that surround my place.

Mental Push-Ups

Trying to get up
Trying to get out
Pop a few pills in my mouth
This one will work no doubt
The pain in my back is gone
(and so is my brain)
So what's left is an emotional train
On the track
Off the track
Up and down
Fast or slow
Recovery is not a perfect straight road
But an end is in sight or so I'm told
To hold, hold, hold and hold on to the rope,
The rope of hope
Get up!
Be up!
Stay up!
Look up!
Thank the One up.

Still on Pins and Needles

Still on pins and needles
Sipping on roots and leaves
Oriental yin yang cleaning

European physical therapy
Cool water swims, ice pack, then
Therapeutic 98 degree water hanging gym

Walking, rolling my back and forth on tennis balls
Praying, meditating, searching for the meaning of it all
Reiki, painting water colors fill my mind
Trying my best to unwind

Relieve, divert the pain in my back and behind
My mind is stretched thin
strong spirit deep within
Out bellows a song from my heart
"GET UP!" time to make a new start.
"GET UP!" time to make your mark.

How Do I Overcome a Setback?

Haven't you heard?
Have you not learned?
You must be still
Humble
and
Submit to His will.

Chapter 3

Weeding

*"Now he that planteth and
he that watereth are one,
and every man shall
receive his own reward
according to his own labour."*

1 Corinthians 3:8

Recovery Phase

Recovery phase
I've arrived through patience and God's mercy, grace
Oh so many months ago sadness and pain always on my face
My faith wrestled with my doubts, such a disgrace
Turmoil in my head, broken hearted,
but my soul, my spirit dwelled in His Holy place
Wherever I turned,
no matter how much my back burned
no matter how deep the pain, or when I could not move
He Loved me just the same
This love showed in the people that cared for me
at physical therapy Jack, Gonzalo, dear Kathy
at acupuncture Dr. Tate, Dr Wong
and the people who mixed the herbal tea
there are others that help me
at neurology Dr Zayas, Susan and Kathy
at my primary Dr Adams and her assistants
Mom, Janice and Jimmie
This next group is cool
pool pals help me
Pam, Sue, Diane, Carol, Alice and a host of smiling faces I see
I must not forget my friends
blessed with so many, forgive me if your name is not written
I love you just the same
I'm in the recovery phase
these friends journyed with me
Pauline, Lee, Dolores, Chris, Dawna, Marjorie,
Teruko, Cheryl, Sheila, Ann, Carolyn, Cindy,
Rev. Craig, Linda, Richard, Diana, Evelyn, Donna, Catherine, Eileen
Robin saved my hair and Reina rescued me from house work

Thanks to beloved churches Bethel and Olney Street.
Their light shined on me
and finally my family
Husband, sons, Reena, Mya grandbaby, my mom, momma, sisters
Nay and Di, nephews and nieces

all were (or are) part of my recovery
So many people to hug
So many people to love
So many people to thank
Simply give God the praise
for His mercy and His grace

I am in the recovery phase
of healing - healed, I prayed
prayers answered, I got up, rose
from mess to message
I learned the true meaning of psalm 23:
"He maketh me...restores me..surely goodness and mercy
follow me...I will dwell…"
Recovery phase
All is well.

No Pain and No Brain

The pain is gone and so is my brain
These pills go down, last much too long
I forget how it felt to feel strong
Was I wrong?
To take strong pills, instead of deep breathe,
meditate, sit stiff still
Now the pain is gone and so is my brain
The sun is shining, looks like it's going to rain
Doesn't matter
Doesn't make sense
There's no common pattern when your thoughts are nonsense
I'll give you my pain for your brain

Is This Temporary Insanity?
(Dedicated to my beloved husband)

I love you more than I could ever love someone
I love you through the night, morning and noon
I love you when it feels good
I love you until it hurts
I love you when there's no reason to love you
My big brown head moon
Despite my mouth, pain, heartache
I love you just the same
Some call it temporary insanity
I call you my love
God's gift
My husband
My love partner
I love to share the joys, trials, and sorrows together
I love you more than ever.

GET UP!

My oldest son tells me to
"GET UP!"
Time to make a new start
'GET UP!"
Time to make your mark.

Use Your Wings

Use your wings
To rise above
SING
Move those earthly things that get in the way
That cast a dark cloud
on what was once a sunny day

Use your wings
SPREAD
Them high and wide
SOAR
Like an eagle
Then glide softly like a butterfly

Use your wings
Divine SPIRIT
Will keep you moving to a higher place
Mercy, grace, peace and love
SURROUNDS
and
Opens my wings
each morning

New mercies
New beginnings.

Angels in Tunnel Vision
(Dedicated to Mary and Jessica @ RI Imaging)

I'm traveling through the tunnel again
The diagnostic test of my back not my brain
Although it sounds like thunder, lightening and rain
Against a dome shaped window pane
I try to quiet my mind, slow down my racing heart
I mustn't hyperventilate, just slow deep breathe from the start
Then out of nowhere a peaceful voice is heard
It stays with me as I cling to every reassuring word
A few more minutes it will be over
In a second we will be done
The test is completed
The healing has begun
Mary the Technician told me that her
hands and wrists were restored
Said she didn't return to her old job or ways anymore
Mary had new hands, stretched out open hearted, she said
God blessed her with a new life
Teaching science, camp ministries, and part time MRI
She radiates peace and love throughout the MRI tunnel
Jessica, like Mary, is sweetness wrapped in a bundle
A student tech who radiates love and light
How can you work all day and
be such a beam of happiness tonight?
Mary and Jessica
MRI queens
Angels in tunnel vision.

Give Thanks

We must not wait to say THANKS
We mustn't hold our breath
when someone takes the time
to lift you up or give you a break
Make no mistake
This can't wait
Just stop, look, smile and say THANKS
Listen to your heart
Obey the voice within
Think about giving thanks
and from the start
Do your part
A smile
A warm hug
A kiss
A soft hand on a broken heart
A smooth stroke on a weak back
Silence
A look
A listening ear
Uninterrupted time
Just being there
A comforting smooth voice
Your choice
not by force
Just loving to love
To share
Give a care
Loving to be me
God's grace and mercy
Is all I need
So I give thanks to the One above
Give thanks, spread cheer and love.

Neurological Sense
(Dedicated to Dr. V. Zayas., Neurologist and Susan Rodrigues)

You have the nerve
To care
To transmit affection
To sit, listen and stare
To feel my pain and respond so sincere

You have the nerve
To stretch beyond your appointment schedules
To take the time to see me again
To ease my mind
To relieve the pain and tension in my spine

You have the nerve
To connect with me
To understand my needs and my longing
To be pain free of this back pain
that has stolen some of my abilities

You have the nerve
To be kind and remind me
that it will take time,
but, eventually
I will be fine

You have the nerve
and compassion for healing

Words are the least way of revealing my thanks
and my warm response
to treatments that flow through every nerve pathway
and every cell
That makes me know that
one day I will be well.

Words are the least way of revealing my thanks
and my warm response
to treatments that flow through every nerve pathway
and every cell
That makes me know that
one day I will be well.

Looking Forward to Going Back

Looking forward to going back
Although pain lingers
in my leg and back
I can no longer worry
or let it hold me back
I must get back to work again
I must listen to my body
and the voice within
Stay calm and treat my spine
as my best friend
Support, strength, flexibility, stretch,
adjust, align, lie down and rest,
stand still, deep breathe, and pray each and every day,
for continued healing and relief of pain
Look forward to looking back
You've come a long way.

Surrender

Silent
Unleash
Recognize
Reach
Everyone
No matter
Directions
Evolve
Righteousness.

Joys and Pains of Loving Our Sons
(Dedicated to the mothers who have lost a son)

You don't know me
I don't know you
But we know each other because

We are called "Mother"
We love our sons
We hug and praise them one by one
They leave us
Some leave to become more educated
On campus
On the streets or just
On the run
They get caught up in pursuing their dream
At times tangled up
While just trying
To be free
To roam
To be alone on their own
Caught up
Bound up
Before finding their way home

We are called "Mother"
Lovers of our sons
One by one
They leave us
For better
For worse
They leave us by car

Plane, train, arrest or bus
They leave us handcuffed
Or they leave on their own

And then one day they return,
Home or heaven bound
Now don't get me wrong
They are strong
And we are not wrong
For loving our sons
From the time they were born

We are called "Mother"
Unconditional lovers
Of our sons
No matter where
Whatever their life becomes.

Faces in the Flowers

I see your face in the flowers
along the roadside painting
A picture of a brighter tomorrow
Your face smiles
It smells of hope
Your stem stands tall
Petals reach out for me and help me to cope
Your roots firmly grounded
Love and mercy surround me
Fertilize my soul
I'm so blessed to have and hold
You in the palm of my hand
Feel your softness
Smell your sweetness
I close my eyes I feel wonderfully blessed
Despite my own mess
I get your positive messages
I am transformed from my mess to message
I am comforted by the energy you send
From the beginning of the day until the end
You have been a loyal and trusted friend
I see your face in the marigolds, pansies,
Roses and chrysanthemums
I thank God for all of you
My dear friends.

South of Heaven
North of Hell

I'm living South of heaven and North of hell
My address depends on my attitude and actions as well

South of heaven
North of hell
Stuck in the middle
Searching for my story
A testimony to tell

South of heaven
North of hell
It's not about me
I've nothing to sell
It's about God's
LOVE...PRAISE...WORSHIP
Feeling so good makes me dance
A HALLELUJAH YELL
Because for now I'm

South of heaven
North of hell
Moving up
Going up
Feeling up
Heading less
South of heaven
More North of hell.

111

What If I Believe
That I'm Pain Free?

I believe I'm there or at least near
The end of my pain
My sufferings over
Don't you hear the silence?
Softness in my voice?
No groaning
No whining
No moaning
Pain is gone
Can I be wrong?
Maybe I just don't think the same
Healing words command my thoughts
Deep breathe
Be present
Have faith
Pray is what I've been taught
Slow the mind
Calm the spirit
Yoga your body
Don't worry if you're behind
Don't quit
Your life depends on it
Take time
Unwind
Catch the flow of new energy
It's free
It's yours
It's mine.

Snowed In

Snowed in
Homebound
Forced to rest again
Listen to what I have learned
about rest, silence, comfort this painful burning back
back up, months ago it was much worse than that
so yes I've come a long way
no need to complain
I've come a long way
even though there's still pain.

Healing Inch-by-Inch

I'm healing inch-by-inch
Mercy by mercy
At times it so small
I can hardly feel any difference at all
But, when I think about His Mercies and Grace
About His promises to me,
I erase all doubts, instead
I keep the faith
That one day I will be healed from this pain, sickness
I'll have strength to run the race
So I press forward to the mark
Of a higher calling
Inhale the Light
See the Light
Feel the Light
Walk in the Light
Without falling
I'm healing inch-by-inch
New mercies
Strong faith within.

Blessings

1 cup worth of pain
Think about what you have gained
1 pound of faith
Think about how far you came
1/2 teaspoon of humility
Think about all your new abilities
1 pinch of mercy
A dash of grace
Think about your blessings each day.

My Parents' Enduring Love

He had so much love that he endured so much pain
My dad
The greatest of the great born in 1928
Oldest son of a farmer and a mom who nursed him
until he was almost eight
They always prayed hard, often prayed late
Always began each day with prayer and thanks
My dad raised his family the same way
His life full of joy and much pain toward the end
He endured so much illness, more than I can comprehend
Blindness, failed kidneys, double amputee
All due to poorly controlled diabetes
His life would be my testimony of pain and suffering
A threshold for physical endurance, an awakening
To the knowledge of what the human body can take
When prayer is the center and in everything give thanks
My mom's life is a lesson in endurance as well
Perseverance and determination is what her story would tell
"Improve on your best," She would hardly let us kids rest
There was so much to learn, so much to see
Time could not be wasted on complaints and worries
Just do it before it is too late
"Do it before someone else takes your place"
My mom's advice and spirit serves us well
At seventy two she's had more than her share of
deaths and sickness too.
So what I've learned are ingredients for success
That's why these writings are
Messages instead of stories about a Mess.

Awaiting Graduation Day

I'm sitting on the threshold
of graduation day
Soon to be released from physical therapy
My progress makes me so happy
Because never have I stuck with an exercise
program for this long and now despite some pain
I feel so much stronger

I'm sitting on the threshold
of graduation day
Thanking God for the Rhode Island Rehabilitation
I've come a long, long way.

Centering My Thoughts

I'm in the center of a field
Gazing at a blue light
Thinking that one day an end will be in sight
The green field is my vision
Gives me hope beyond reason
The golden rays of the sun
Reminds me there are more roads to run
It's not over
I've just begun to taste peace
To taste relief

I am teased by this feeling
This sensation of profound healing
Validating my faith
Strengthening my belief
That God is all around me
In the field
In the sky,
In my every breath
In my mind

I'm in the center of a field
Gazing at a blue light
Thinking, knowing that one day soon
A bright and shining end is in sight.

Dr. Chopra
(Dedicated to Pradeep Chopra MD)

Did you say your name is Chopra
Like (as in) Deepak Chopra
Any relations?
I felt like I was part of a sting operation
Another needle to my spine
But I was sure this time that it would be my last
Or at least the thought of surgery was in the distant past

He assured me he could help me
I've heard that many times
I put my faith foot forward
Tried my best to unwind
As He put the needle deep into my spine
What a relief I felt
Anesthetized spine
Instant relief
Comfort beyond belief
But for only a few days
Okay,
Dr. Chopra
Try it another way
Your reputation, kind words and smiles
are enough to make my return worth the while.

Chapter 4

Reaping

"For we are labourers together with God:
ye are God's husbandry,
ye are God's building."

1 Corinthians 3:9

Feeling Free

I'm at the end of 2003
Feeling mentally and spiritually free
No one left to forgive
Let go of all hateful thoughts
between you and me
2003 filled with struggles to relieve my back pain
But through God's grace and mercy
I grew
I gained
More faith and patience silenced my suffering
I learned to remain steadfast
Unmoved, standing, praying, resting and relaxing
Accepting help, advice
Temporary limitations
Stepping back

Stepping out in faith
Moving forward, looking toward 2004
Full healing, strength, growth, secure

Stepping out in faith
Running, jumping, praising,
forgave and forgiven
free of hate.

Leaning On My Father's Cane

Did I know that once again I would lean on you
and that you would prop me up, propel my legs forward too
support my spine, encourage me each time
I threatened to just fall back
give up and let the pain engulf my mind
My father's cane a piece of him after he died
I kept this cane, often hugged it and at times kept it by my side
Little did I know that I would depend on it
Depend on hearing dad's voice, see his face, just a bit
Feeling the smooth, firm, warmth of his cane
walking with me, easing my pain
Reminiscing his love for me again
I bear down and strain to hear
his messages whispered in my ear:
"Don't worry, the fat lady hasn't sung
it's not over, you've just begun
rest, pray, don't be tempted to run
slow down, hear yourself breath
stretch your arms and hands out, feel the coolness of the breeze
as sure as the sun shines, know that you will be healed
mind, body, soul, spirit
rest, pray even after healing is done."

How Is Your Back?

My back is not all of me
Instead of flowers
people are sending me advice and remedies
Today I received
a box of arthritis joint patches
for use on my back, neck and extremities

I've been told I should take up a hobby like quilting
I didn't know that my body would be
the first try of my artistic abilities
I'm wearing four patches for pain
Each patch different
but their goals are the same

One for deep nerve pain
One for superficial burning pain
One for muscle and joint aches
One to warm me up so I can exercise
Makes my hips shake

My body looks like a quilt
My spirit is a quilt of all
the people in my life
who care to see me well.

Back-to-Back Poems

Back-to-back poems
about my back
about triumph and pain
Much talk about what I gained
in the past year
it's clear to me
that I must start each day
with God near
Here in my mind
in my heart
right from the start
dawning of each new day
stop, breathe, meditate and pray
and if inspired, spirit filled
write a poem or short story if you will
back-to-back poems
standing high on my toes
moving forward
towards
the goal
healing, healed
peace, tranquility
inside out with God
hear, here, it's clear
He must be everywhere
where I am
everywhere
with you and
where we walk and stand.

125

The Upper Room

In the upper room
I am consumed
by the White Light
that shines so bright
on the crown of my head
straight down to my toes
only God knows
the thoughts in my mind
at this time

So heavenly, so rich
I can hardly feel the itch
of this spider on my arm
oblivious to any harm
that is near me
because I'm protected
by the very Light I see
surrounded by peace
warmed by peace
warmed by love
embraced by the Holy Spirit
from above.

Potpourri Care

Pins and needles
heat, massage, ice
light beams

Ointments, creams
water, ice pack coolers
whirlpool heat

Inspiring words
chocolate chip cookie treats

Potpourri of care
like a wild dream
and a nightmare

It's all good

Everything has happened
(for a reason)
No fear, as it should.

A Journey Back

I'm on a journey back
Picking up the pieces
of the gold that I left behind
Tracing my steps
as I back track
Remembering each time
I fell
Got back up
Wrote a poem
A story to tell

You and me
Don't give up!
Stand up!
Push back!
Away!
Push up!
At times be quiet!
Shut up!
Look up!
Raise your hands up!
Feel the spirit
Move up and down your spine
You're on your way back
To moving up again.

My Conversation with God

"I'm here, sitting right in your brain
It's as if you're riding in a train
Sit back!
Relax!
Refrain from worry!
Look at the facts!
If you abide in Me and I in you
There is no limit to what you can do
But if you're fearful and uncertain every day
Without faith, you will never find your way
My opinion is that you
Rest in Me
Stay!
Dwell!
Abide!
Show some love!
Pray!
Trust Me to give you the right words to say
Trust me to make everything okay
At the end of your journey
You'll thank Me and sing praise
I'll thank you and say well done
Faithful servant
You obeyed
Now come!"

MIA - Missing in Action

Out of sight
Out of mind
Waiting
Hoping
Hurting
But now I'm
Out of time
Too late to return
Too far away from what I learned
Once I could do double the amount
of my work
and yours too
Now I must focus on the good
I can do
Go inside
Build up my spirit
Nurture my mind
Focus on the important things in life
Move away from worry
Embrace the words of the Wise
Walk strong
Most of all
Thank God for my life.

Praise - Exercise Song

Stomp your feet
Clap your hands
Sing God's glory all over this land

Raise your voice
Look up to the sky
Praise His name
you got to shout and rejoice

Turn to the right
Hold your head up high
Wave your arms side to side
Feel the spirit inside

Say thank you Jesus
Thank you Christ
Thank you Lord
You've always been by my side

So we say...
Stomp your feet
Clap your hands
Sing God's glory all over this land.
(repeat verses)

The End of the Beginning

When does it end?
It ends when the praise begins
When you thank God for pain
and release all anger within

When does it end?
When shall I put down my pen?
It ends when you stop waiting
for the pain to begin again

How shall I know
if this is the last one?
If this is the last back pain poem
About my journey through back pain
Although I'm still not the same

Neither is a seed
that's had sun and rain
Neither are its flowers
a sign that it's the end
It begins and ends over and over again
It's all over when praise is deep within

Like the seed in rich soil, buried deep, out of sight
We need that special oil in our body,
so our lamp shines bright
Don't worry when it ends or when it begins
Focus on the healing light within.
'Cause it's over as soon as the praise begins.

One Year Ago

One year ago You called me,
whispered in my ear
Lie down, rest and stay here
Write whatever I tell you
Erase all fear
Don't worry about dotted I's or crossed T's

Just listen closely to Me
I'll tell you what to write
The words will flow faster
than a beam of light
and when you've finished each poem
You'll know I've been with you
from morning to dawn

Comforting words
to soothe your soul
Spirit filled thoughts
to make you whole
Heal your body, mind and spirit
To ease the pain,
So follow Me
Don't quit.

A Year of Thanks

Pauline, Chris, Teruko, Judy, Lee
Carolyn, Dolores, Ann, Naomi
You've been with me along with my family

True loyal friends stuck by me
Not just off and on, you stayed consistently

Visits, telephone calls, encouraged me
to see a brighter day
When I was too filled with pain to say
I know I'll get there
come what may

There were times all I wanted to do was lay
in bed, hide my head, turn away but,
you pulled the covers down
helped me up, turned me around

You wouldn't let go until my feet were on the ground
So, I thank you for one year
Thank God for you and for always being there.

Wake Up!

Wake up, Wake up, Wake up
Sharp pokes in my back, buttocks and legs
Please let me sleep I beg

Wake up, wake up, and wake up
I open my eyes but still in a daze
This whole thing is enough to make you feel crazed

Why is this pain arresting me, holding me hostage this day
Waking me, stealing my peace
at this hour today

Wake up, wake up, and wake up
my attention is open and clear
I will not fear because God is near
But this pain is enough to make one fear

The worst that could happen is not more than I can bear
The worst that could happen is that I would forget that God is
always here

Wake up, wake up, and wake up
The pain alarm sounds
Attention! pain makes me listen
to the rhythm of my heart beat sounds

makes me listen to my breath
Makes me listen to Divine
Makes me listen to all the spiritual messages all around.

Happy Birthday, Cleo!

I'm fifty, I'm fifty
I'll never forget
The Blessings that God has in store for me yet
I'm fifty, I'm fifty
I'll never forget
The Blessings that God has in store for me yet.

Can You Help Me?

"I can't help you"
What the surgeon said was true
Yet, I serve a God that will see me through
the bad times and the good
what may look like the end
is really the start of something new
"I can't help you"
is partially true
because you've helped me to ask God, "Now, what am I to do ?"
Turn your head, push your faith foot forward, and move,
Keep on praying, dwell, and listen silently,
Help is coming sooner than eventually.

The Pain
Will Not Hurt You Anymore

The pain will not hurt you anymore
Hang in, there's more blessings for you in store

Press, press, you must not get depressed
Press and rest

Find the balance between what is real,
in the unseen
and what you've seen
between

What it is that you feel
and what it all means

Press, press, rest and press
More faith
Trust in the Lord
Your pain will not hurt you anymore.

Who Am I?

I am more than my back
I have a mind, heart, spirit and soul
I have the Divine love living in my bones

I am more than my back
There is nothing that I lack
Other than relief
and
at times a belief
that I will run again
without feeling pain
But, I am alright
I'm more than what's in your sight

I am more than my back
Painful as it is, I am here still
Determined and strong willed
I am living according to God's will.

Going Back and Moving Forward

I am going back to physical therapy
But, nothing seems the same
It's really like a boot camp for back pain

You can moan and groan through each stretch
Still you must keep up with the reps
You can grit your teeth
and search for relief
But, the stretches you must still repeat

A burning back, a shaky left leg
Sweat pouring down my forehead
Lifting a ten pound brick of lead
I'd rather be at home in my bed

It all seems so insane
Weight lifting with back pain,
I'll either lose or gain
strength, flexibility, control of my back pain.

Welcome Back

I'm back to being home
I have a comfort level that I hadn't known,
For so many months I lived outside of myself
Due to daily doses of pain, I forgot how good relief felt
This sudden relief of my painful burning back
After trying a method I accepted on faith
Despite initial excruciating pain
never the less I was urged to allow the therapists to train
me into a new frame of mind
"to work through the pain," they said and "soon relief I will
find,"
I gingerly held the course
I surrendered, submitted to protocol
because the Lord promised me, I would have relief from it all
The Lord promised me that I would be made well
Now, severe back pain, leg pain is part of my past
Through prayer, mindful exercise, thank God, this relief will last.

What Is Faith?

You know that the sun is up there
although today it has not appeared

You know the wind is part of the air
yet you've never seen it, you feel its presence all around here

You know the fragrance resembles a rose
yet you look around and there are no flowers before your nose

You know the warm touch of love
but, yet you refuse to acknowledge the Holy One above

You know that the trees turn green,
what a magnificent gorgeous scene

You know that the flowers bloom,
grapes grow as large as mushrooms,
without a gardener and without ever being pruned

You feel your heart beat
regardless of what you think and understand
you hear the soft voice of a sweet command

You call it your instincts, your gut, your master wit
but, yet your intelligent self won't thank God for all of it.

Holy Spirit, Move through the Pain

Pain can be your best friend
If you let the Holy Spirit in
If you don't worry about if you win
If you believe, obey, surrender to God
Call upon the risen King

Pain can be your best friend
It will make you stop whatever you're doing
Pain will force you to start your life all over again
A new direction
A new song
Putting you on the track where you belong

Pain can be your best friend
Making you lie down in green pastures
Making you look up
Pray to the Master
"Have mercy on me Lord
I'm ready to begin
I'm ready to accept Christ, His pain, His resurrection
His living Spirit,
He's my friend."

Stripped Down

Stripped down
Naked
Pain patches off
I'm not afraid
Just shivering even though
The weather temperature is 94
Nose running
Stomach upset
Yawning
Craving
For relief, for my percocet
Stripped down
Naked
I can make it
Clean out
Cleaned within
But, here comes the intense burning pain again
Oh, how I want to give in and
start the narcotic analgesic again
Sweat pouring off my brow
Seven days of restlessness
what a mess
And then peace comes
like a cool breeze
oh, what?... some relief.

Why So Much Pain?

Why so much pain?
Why so much suffering?
Perhaps it's time to stop
Stop the questions and complaints
Who am I to question God?
Who am I to challenge God's wisdom?
Who am I to blame?
claim injustice,
to act full of my self, to be so vain?

Now I have eyes of faith
Fearful and in awe
at such a great
God, Mighty God, Sovereign God
Everything under heaven is His
Oh, now my eyes see what my ears have heard
I finally get it I finally learn
God has power over ALL things
My faith is now strengthened, strong
I CAN carry on
Suffering and pain is no longer a heavy load of questions
No longer a sack of complaints or demanding expectations
God caught my attention
He rescued me from myself
I humbly bow down in submission
confessing and repenting
I accept His will and no one else's
I take a deep breath
and let it out
I'm ready for a brand new start
I got the message loud and clear
Let go and let God
Oh yes, now I hear.

Flying through the Storm

Five birds hover around a huge ocean wave storm

Bird number one just wants to dare someone
to fly through the wave
because he's not so brave

Bird number two is too eager to know
the dangers ahead
so without much thought he goes

Bird number three would rather wait and see
if the other bird makes it through this dangerous journey

Bird number four flies high above it all
He doesn't want to ruffle his feathers or risk having a fall

Bird number five joyfully blazes the sky on the other side
Has he already been through the storm and survived?

Remember Me

Remember Me
As you walk your life journey
Remember Me with each breath,
With each sign, with each step
Remember Me when your feet feel heavy,
When the road feels rough
Remember Me when the going gets tough
Remember Me as you step up and step out,
Remember that serving and praising Me is what it's all about
Remember Me when you miss a step, slip and fall
Remember Me through it all
As you reach for My Hand, hold on grip the bar,
pull yourself up, again, you've come much too far
Remember Me when you just want to stand and
Wait on the step because you don't understand
Remember Me when your steps take a wrong turn,
Remember there's always something that you must learn,
Remember Me when you come to the end,
Remember there's always a new step to begin
Remember Me now, remember Me when
remember I, God, am with you
Through thick and thin.

*"Call upon me in the day of trouble: I will deliver thee,
and thou shalt glorify me."*

Psalm 50:15

FROM MESS TO MESSAGE

Cleo Darcia Graham, NP

About the Book

What if a sudden injury or illness changed your life leaving you feeling helpless and confused - in a big mess?

What if you asked God to heal you?

What if you asked God to help you get through the pain and suffering?

What if He answered, but not in the way that you expected?

Read Cleo Darcia Graham's poetic collection of her conversations with God, including inspirational messages of hope, that testify to the power of prayer. Clearly, the author is a witness to the connection between mind, body, and spiritual healing as a means of self-renewal and renewed devotion to God.

From Mess to Message - *Understanding the Hidden Healing Messages Behind Pain and Suffering* is a must read for anyone who is trying to find their way back to health.

About the Author

Cleo Graham, RNP, BSN, MN, is a Board Certified Nurse Practitioner and Holistic Health Counselor who has worked over twenty- five years as a clinician and educator. She graduated from Adelphi University, Columbia University and the University of Rhode Island. She was a recipient of the American Heart Association - NE Affiliate Nurse of the Year Award in 2000. As a Director of Women's Ministry, she leads group meetings for her church family.

She wrote this book during her own battle through pain and suffering after a sudden back injury that changed her life. Although she received skillful medical care and integrated holistic treatment, she knew that physical healing was not enough to mend the emotional stress and trauma. Once she surrendered herself to the Higher Power, she immediately grew more connected to the Lord and she was blessed to receive His answers swiftly. She listened with a spiritual ear and humbly recorded these answers from God. The result of her total submission and reliance on God is now an important literary work revealing a divinely inspired journey.

A Note From the Author

I would like to thank you for taking the time to read **From Mess To Message** - *Understanding the Hidden Healing Message Behind Pain and Suffering*. It is my hope that you understand the hidden healing message behind pain and suffering, and that you are comforted in knowing that there is a higher path toward health.

I welcome your comments.

Be Blessed Always,

> Cleo D. Graham, NP
> cleograham@aol.com
> P.O. Box 14473
> East Providence, R.I. 02914

Order Page

From Mess to Message
Understanding the hidden healing messages behind pain and suffering

$14.97 + 2.50 (S&H)

Visit us online at:
www.BooksToBelieveIn.com

Phone:
(303) 794-8888

Fax:
(720) 863-2013

Mail:
**Thornton Publishing, Inc.
17011 Lincoln Ave. #408
Parker, Colorado 80134**

If books are temporarily sold out at your favorite bookstore, have them order more of **ISBN: 1-932344-89-6**

Name: _____

Address: _____

_____

Phone: _____

E-mail: _____

Credit Card #: _____

Card Type: _____ (Visa, Mastercard, American Express, Discover)

Security Code: _____ Expiration Date: ____/____